Folding the Crane
POEMS

June 1st, '02

To Kevin + Jennifer:

Thank you both for your support.

May your days
be filled with
vibrant
rainbows.

Always!

J. Andres Luna

Folding the Crane

POEMS

T. Anders Carson

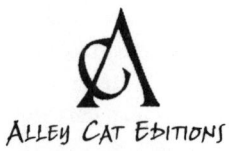

ALLEY CAT EDITIONS

Copyright © 2002 by T. Anders Carson

All rights reserved. No part of this publication may be reproduced or transmitted in any form or by any means, electronic or mechanical, including photocopying, or any information storage and retrieval system without a licence from CANCOPY (Canadian Copyright Licensing Agency), 1 Yonge Street, Suite 1900, Toronto, Ontario, Canada, M5E 1E5.

These poems have appeared in full or in part in the following publications: The Brobdingnagian Times (IRL), Convergence (CAN), The Cracked Mirror (US), Crystal Drum (US), Dialogue Among Civilizations Through Poetry (UN), freefall (US), Intangible (CAN), The Journal (UK), Mocambo (CAN), Nerve Cowboy (US), Parlor Games and Other Eccentricities (IND), Pegasus (US), Poetry Motel (US), Sepia (UK), and Shine (IND).

Canadian Cataloguing in Publication Data

Carson, T. Anders
Folding the crane: poems

ISBN 1-894498-03-8

I. Title.

PS8555.A7725F64 2002   C811'.54   C2002-900602-3
PR9199.3.C425F64 2002

The publisher gratefully acknowledges the Canada Council for the Arts for its support of our publishing program.

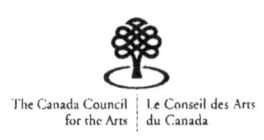

The Canada Council   Le Conseil des Arts
for the Arts   du Canada

Alley Cat Editions
an imprint of Boheme Press
382 Briston Private, Lower Suite
Ottawa, Ontario, Canada K1G 5R2
www.bohemeonline.com

For Victoria,
I believe . . .

Folding the Crane

It is a Japanese tradition that if you fold 1000 origami cranes that your wish will come true. In Los Alamos, New Mexico, I came across a children's book relaying the story of young Sadako, a Hiroshima survivor. Her goal was to fold the necessary cranes in order for her "sickness" to end. Unfortunately she died before she could complete the task. Her classmates finished the collection and set up a monument in Peace Park. The statue in Hiroshima reads: *This is our cry, this is our prayer. Peace in the world.* The poems in this collection suggest the urgency and strata of hope that is necessary for survival. I draw on the strength needed to overcome crisis and seek stillness in the wailing pace of living. These poems are my humble origami cranes that I'm folding in honour of Sadako's ebullient vision.

Table of Contents

CLAW

Let it Come	13
Beneath a Trembling Branch	15
On the Road to Los Alamos	17
Back at the Hammer Again	19
Crawling through Spiked Borders	21
Where Did You Go, My Son?	23
Juggling the Children	24
How to Make an Entrance	25
A Reminiscent Tear	27
A December Cloud	28
Alone in a Café in Paris	29
Beyond Stillness	31

BREAST
I

Six Haikus	35
I Saw a Room	36
A Grape	37
Unwaking the Almost Dead	38
An Impatient Bark	40
Burning Grass	41
Things that are Wonderful	42
In a Moment's Breath	43
Continental Breakfast	44

BREAST
II

Sorrow	47
A Basket of Distress	49
Fallen Angel	50
It is Morning	51
A Silent Phone	53
I Can Smile	55
A Sunday Afternoon	56
Pink Fluorescent Legs	57

WINGS

Under a Blue Sheet	61
Maternity Leave	62
Daisy Filled with Tears	63
In the Office	64
Awaiting Children	65
A Child's Heartbeat	66
For Emilia	67
Pulling a Sleigh	68
In a Chinese Buffet	69
A Soother in my Pocket	71
My Daniel	72
An Eagle's Wing	74
Quest for Absolution	75
Singing the Song	76

Claw

Darkness reigns
at the foot of the lighthouse.

— *Japanese proverb*

LET IT COME

This meaning that exists within all of us.
This undying pain that circles our most sensitive areas.
It is only when regions of sanity are located,
when grassfires have been extinguished,
when the sea has been poisoned by nuclear tests,
that we finally see the madness that quells itself
inside our very selective vision.
When you have an NRA rifle range the size of small countries
at the top of New Mexico.
When you've completed all detonations above ground for kicks.
You realize the small trailer homes that are swept away in cyclones
or tornadoes or hurricanes are really our own endangered lives
when we wish the destruction of each other.
Let it come.
This day of remorse and remembrance.
This day of raising flags at half mast
and playing the final notes to Taps.
This day of saying why must they suffer those radiation tears?
Why must they roll in fires of hatred
and drown in the protection of water?
This is the day.
Let it come.
Let it come when they are busy watching *Nightline*,
or checking the stock market,
or signing a new mortgage for that dream home.
Let it come.
Let it seep into the dreams of our children
so that they awake from this fantastic nightmare.
That it keeps us from sleeping,
those distant cries.
Not even earplugs can hold back angst.
Not even the saturated newspaper with clips of yesterday's shooting.
Not even the revelation of another sexual position
that the President has helped himself to.
Let it come.
It will erupt like a plague.

It will corrupt the young and help the old.
This is coming.
Get your coffee ready.
Add some cream and a dash of sugar.
Get your K-Mart chair.
Sit outside your humble house,
put your feet on the barbecue,
and just watch the sky for colours.

Beneath a Trembling Branch

The eyes often believe what they see –
that is why it is fluid in its sanctity.
It can follow the proper flow of water.
Not watching the way it can absolve truth
and impertinent dissidence.
I can remember a time
when all the leaves once grew,
and that none were stunted by acid rain
or the onslaught of an early Spring.
I can remember when our wells used to be full
and we didn't have to revert to old rituals
for the water to flow.
I can remember when gasoline was abundant
and it bubbled from the ground.
Now it is fought over by armies
and guerilla warfare.
The means to torture,
burning crosses of oilfields in effigy.
I can remember when children didn't fear the sky;
they would look up at it
as if it were a blanket
that a parent was going to use to tuck them in.
Today it is a surging fear
that radiates from those awestruck eyes.
Is this the bombing that will begin the end?
I can remember when water was fresh and clean and good.
It didn't make you sick.
It didn't make daddy sick.
It didn't give mommy the lump on her breast.
What happened?
Why the infusion of waste upon the dismembered,
low end, multi-racial supposed water-seekers?
Why?
So that profits can rise
and share prices can balloon.
I didn't know that a branch could hold so much.

I didn't think that it was strong enough for this weight.
The little bird of alchemy
sits on a solitary branch
and plays solitaire,
singing softly and wistfully to the breeze.
Only in that repetitive action
will life become clear.
It will fold into a fresh tree;
an origami of the mind.
I know that this branch must be allowed to grow.
It must.
For within its tiny bud
lies humanity as thin as a butterfly's wing.
It rolls in ancient prayers.
It fasts in deserts until clarity is released.
The clouds of watering favour
flow over the abundant fields.
Grow my little branch,
hold the limbs of torture.

On the road to Los Alamos

I lost my way.
I hadn't talked to the secret men in black coats
to tell them my purpose.
They thought I was a Russian,
or possibly German,
but I fooled them because
I am Canadian.
At least today I am.
This doesn't help when you try
to get up to the site where it all started –
the making of the gadget to stop the war;
the continuation of struggling minds
to find more concise ways of killing our fellow man.
It is far more humane to just poison the water,
but they like to have these big blasts.
These big feelings of domination and superiority.
This all happened on my way to Los Alamos.
I did find it.
I found it up the sloping road
that winds itself into oblivion.
You feel as if you are going to the top of the world.
Trucks use the entire plethora of gears.
But what I found in the bookstore in Los Alamos,
the one beside the museum to commemorate science's greatest
achievement:
I found a book for a child.
It should be required reading for all of us;
not just the latest score
or Wall Street madness.
I see the way it is.
I can see it.
A story about a child in Hiroshima;
the story you don't want to remember.
The children.
Sure, you look with a sense of awe
when mushrooms float up into the sky,

but what about the tears of this child?
And the many other children that have cried
at the madness that comes from combat,
both physical and mental.
I don't see a vision.
Maybe I lack the gorge sight
of the most brilliant Ph.D.,
but I do know that when money
is being put towards these programs of death,
children will ultimately suffer.
It is fine to think of yourself and that retirement;
that you deserve this after so many years of work.
But it is the children who will have to clean this up.
They will see the flash
and if we are not careful,
they will be gone.

Back at the Hammer Again

I have traveled 2500 miles to come here.
I have visited the grave of Elvis.
He wasn't in.
He was busy watching old footage of the Trinity Site explosion.
He choked on his peanut butter and banana sandwich.
It was toasted just so.
I crossed the Mississippi River and then sat in traffic
for over an hour.
The back-up was fierce into Memphis.
Both bridges were clogged.
I watched the dial of my car.
Creeping along at less than two miles an hour,
delta blues ringing in my speakers.
I knew it must be a bad one.
At last,
people getting the great rubber neck.
Pieces of flesh lying on the Interstate.
Grim State Troopers carefully moving traffic.
Two aid workers holding up a green blanket
as the torched semi and car lie in charred silence.
It took me awhile to recover.
I wondered about the blanket,
why it wasn't white.
I guessed that stains are easily hidden amongst
the wonderful shades of the military.
I stopped at the Welcome Center,
relieved myself in ancient Arkansas urinals,
and watched the lady answer touristic questions.
Most wanted cheap prices of motels
but all had to tell somebody, anybody
about the gruesome horror
we all had faced.
She became an analyst listening quietly,
nodding her head at the appropriate times.
Shaking it at others.
I thanked her from all of us.

I thanked her for listening to our own little internal hells
that had followed us off the turnpike –
those that take the right at the next light;
those that pull up to the next drive-thru.
All she said was:
You cope . . .
I wouldn't until further on.
It wasn't until the next day
that I saw a speeding vehicle behind me;
she was breathing heavily.
He was holding the foot to the floor.
I knew that speed.
I knew the reason for four-way flashers
without snow or rain.
A baby was coming.
Within two days,
I witnessed the last face of death
and the crawling fear of birth –
they both ride the same foregoing line.

Crawling through Spiked Borders

Pushing the dingy button,
cough of: "Yes, we are in.
Who would you like to see?"
"Why, my brother of course."
"I am sorry . . .
He is currently busy passing stools
in front of friends.
He's watching urine puddles pile the corridor
and cigarette butts sullenly drown.
He can't see you right now,
as he is on suicide watch,
filled in a cell full of terror and longing."
Camera motions every movement.
Carefully sliding
as he tries to masturbate to sleep.
You can't be too careful.
"He can't see you right now
as guards are carefully searching his anus
for lost diamonds and packets of concealed cocaine.
He can't see you right now,
'cause he's urinating publicly in a cup
to check the toxicity of his soul.
He can't see you right now,
as handcuffs are folded neatly folded
behind his back.
I'm sure you're aware
he's in prison attire.
He can't see you right now,
'cause he's in the middle of a game of bridge,
playing for the high stakes of cigarettes
and channel choices.
He can't see you right now
because he's in a corner
crying over the loss of parents,
freedom, and sanity.
He doesn't need to be disturbed.

The doctor will soon be in
to give him that sedative.
We find that it helps relax the inmates.
He can't see you right now
because you're obviously trying to help
and that would eventually put us out of business,
so you can just sit down and wait your turn.
We tend to give preference
to mother's praying
and small infants.
We find it fills the thick glass with a mist.
He can't see you right now
but rest assured,
we'll let him know
that you were in."

Where did you go, my son?

You boarded that plane
with the fight and spirit
of a battered child.
You wrote me a letter from the front,
addressed it to mom;
homesickness so apparent in your few words.
I knew you were suffering.
You didn't tell of the torn skin
or lost minds that you were witnessing;
it was only about how your were going to come back
and help build your mom a home.
That home was never built.
I received your letter yesterday.
It came from a friend of yours.
It wasn't too late to remember.
I can see your face,
the tears stream down my cheeks.
I want to hold you again, my son;
I want the twenty years that I had with you
to mean something.
All I have left is a medal in a drawer
and your name far away
on a black wall in Washington.

Juggling the Children

I have seen the divorced juggle children.
They can sometimes throw them high in the air.
But that usually unbalances things
and children fall,
breaking arms and hearts.
I've seen a small group juggle.
Intensity is great;
they must focus on those flailing arms,
legs, and hair.
It works for awhile,
then concentration is lost;
again arms and legs break
and those tiny hearts.
There are some who believe
that if you teach children to juggle themselves,
they will be able to cope admirably.
I watch for these children
as they fling themselves in the air,
hoping and secretly wishing
that the arms of an elder
will catch their frenzied fall.

How to make an entrance

You call yourself a doctor.
Deliver numerous babies
with the help of colleagues,
sign your name at the bottom
of birth certificates.
You rub oils of solitude on the elderly
and prescribe antibiotics to parrots with the flu.
You administer cholesterol tests on the weary
forcing them into a life filled with Melba Toast
and unsalted peanuts.
Whatever happened to the societal look of justice
when seen through a trusting physician's eyes?
Whatever happened to all of those dollars that went
to The Jerry Lewis Telethon?
Whatever happened to the one-legged man
taking on Canada one step at a time?
Whatever happened to the faith that was present
in both schools and families?
Whatever happened to those good times
from the stock market?
Whatever happened to greasy oil changes
that seemed like they were done only yesterday?
Whatever happened to Friday bank line-ups
for weekend money?
Whatever happened to the belief in both languages?
Whatever happened to job security?
Whatever happened to Ben Johnson?
Whatever happened to innocent until proven guilty?
What happens to all of that dead time?
Whatever happened to our lakes filled with countless fish?
Whatever happened to the rain forest in British Columbia?
Whatever happened to bug zappers killing all insects?
Whatever happened to 1984?
Whatever happened to JFK?
What happened in that last pullout at Saigon?
Whatever happened to all of those kids on Ritalin?

Whatever happened to the suicide statistics in Canada?
I know.
She uses surgical gloves to cover up pieces
of a carefully displaced body.
She is on the coroner's report
in every one of us
and the verdict,
upon further review;
yet, another one of our citizens
has slipped and fallen dead
in a tub.

A REMINISCENT TEAR

Rocking towards the curl
of a Northern wind,
Christmas lights on low,
a choral chant echoes
inside dark walls.
A baby clears its throat.
A cat yawns by the fire.
A lover softly breathes
with the help of an English
hot water bottle.
A scene of Christmas:
my father kneeling in front
of a tangled piled of lights,
cancer eating his insides,
calming his hyper disposition.
Threading those lights
with the patience
of a beggar in New Delhi.
There is all but time now.
Unfolding the knot,
the hardened scope of understanding,
his two children afraid to breathe.
He sat there in a fashionable stance
and uncoiled the evil inside.
Sadly the tears had already been shed –
a motion for release.
A striped housecoat;
kneeling on the floor
periodically closing
his stiffening hands –
a fragile crack
fraught with fear.

A December cloud

A wisp of sullen images
varies inside.
It is a controlled stream of suffering.
From the first regal thought
to the jaundiced phase of birth,
it remains.
I know that holidays can crush our spirits;
oppression as thick as High Mass.
A glimmer of reduced mania.
Coy emotions that Christmas morning produces.
Having family scattered to the edges of institutions
is hardening my fears.
It is a loose stool aboard a Greyhound,
or a slight slip off of a frozen runway.
Keep those seat belts on
until you come to a complete stop.
A low level of pressure is present
at cranial temple;
it pumps in time to the sinister scenario
that has been blocked.
One day a key will be produced
and the cobweb horrors that have so faintly
been convinced of reason
shall relegate a shred of destruction.
It is from within that you can see
a December cloud appear.
It arrives in a translucent phrase
and drives the temperature
below recognition.
That December cloud,
full of poison,
struggling paraphernalia,
and hushed prayers.

Alone in a Café in Paris

Tears flowing beyond recognition.
Cold, damp, slightly surreal.
For years fighting the stinging demons
that whisper in the night.
They crawl beneath the covers and
penetrate every stained orifice.
Tears in the Louvre,
not from the magic of art,
but the stale thread of sadness
and loss of sanity.
Crying in a corner.
Mascara running in streams.
The waiter is visibly nervous.
A call is placed.
Three slumbering men,
one carrying a box of oxygen,
as if this tank will fill her lungs with hope.
In the Louvre,
her tears,
a glass of water.
Someone taps her on the shoulder.
Can you breathe?
Yes.
It has nothing to with breathing.
It is lungs collapsing under cancer tents.
It is the creamed kiss of a lover
who will never return.
He is beyond that civil grasp.
He is beyond that fast running Seine.
Please Madame, come with us . . .
Cornered in the Louvre,
a full glass of water with
harried demons still biting her soul.
With my eyes
I ask the waiter
if she is OK.

Les pompiers sont ici maintenant.
They'll never be able to extinguish her burning flame.

Beyond Stillness

Afternoon calm at dusk.
Cat in window purring to the screen.
Tom Waits shielding sorrow
with a dented spoon.
Incense curls from a vein.
A baby sleeps the sleep.
Birds play in last rays of light.
Wind beyond silent.
Sky littered with stars.
Buttering a warm piece of toast.
Sharing it with a lover.
Splitting an organic kiwi.
Size doesn't really matter;
it's how you use it.
Phone is silent.
TV is silent.
The world is silent;
yet, one can still hear
the faint dropping of bombs.

Breast
I

LIVE
to the point of tears.

— *Albert Camus*

Six haikus

January freeze;
body warm under clear tub;
note left unwritten.

Wind blowing leaves;
a bow of lines
form across my face.

A hill full of blossoms;
cows lazily chewing,
alive another day.

Leaving the Interstate;
a row of plastic bags;
carefully blowing.

To see a makeshift shadow,
stumble across room.
Crib is silent; birth is near.

A little girl in tub,
giggles within bubbles,
pointing at dolphins.

I SAW A ROOM

Yesterday,
I saw a room
filled with the laughter of children,
moans of love
and a sunshine sheet.
I saw a room
that was filled with memories
cut without fear.
I saw a room,
added on about twenty years ago,
circling the stages of life.
Fevers battled,
books grippingly read,
thoughts and memories rolling
through the days.
I saw a room
that felt warm yet cold
and whispered the words,
I could get sick here . . .
Nurses on the ready;
windows opened wide;
to let out fear
and welcome the night.

A GRAPE

When a small group of children gather,
there is always a chance mishap; perhaps
a fluke,
a tiny conflagration.
But it does happen.
It did in my small town.
A young boy.
A grape.
Nestled in windpipe.
Shades of frightened purple
and then the look of glass.
Today, tomorrow, and the day after,
his mother will visit the cemetery.
She sees that folded boy's dreams,
can feel his yearning to live.
You can see all of this from across the road.
You are just picking up your car from another tire rotation.
A visitor leaving gifts of supplication
beneath the frail and coloring skin
of an out of season,
crisp, Californian grape.

Unwaking the almost dead

It comes up after a full moon;
this disturbance,
this disruptive sign.
I know it can only mean trouble.
I've tried hard to keep the howling cats apart.
I've tried to understand the secrets of rays upon skin –
radiant rays full of tones of phosphorescence.
I believe that they do need to be awakened.
They who haunt my daily dreams,
hopes,
fears.
They are there beyond the forest,
beyond the set of trails
leading to somewhere;
where the lush grasses have held
the embrace of unhurried lovers;
where the stars have been gazed
by unseen eyes.
I choose a path;
an existence that comes into contact
with this nefarious realm.
The sight of them
makes me lose both appetite and sleep.
The trenchant fear that keeps
a woman awake,
listening for breath at her barred door.
I feel this whisper of anxiety.
It is present when someone unpacks groceries,
filling counters with food
that can no longer be afforded such views.
I pet the stable cat.
She purrs her insolence at me,
her hatred that is everything just and mischievous.
She sits up on the sill
and releases a Sphinx stare.
She looks out over vast desert,

more complete than any ocean,
those eyes of condolence
that have been bitten by sun.

An impatient bark

Cupped with hands of death;
strangled before coffin is lifted;
crawling in a pool of panting blood.
I knew that it would be difficult.
This understanding of ritual violence and neglect.
I knew it would never do
to try and understand it.
It just doesn't.
It could never feel right.
Injustice is far too great a grievance.
It spirals in the stem of the Yucca
and circles in wings of strained crows.
Magpies chuckle at the dogs.
They are not so impatient.
They don't believe in the coming of help;
they just scatter when cars come too close.
They follow the flow of laughter to the skies.
Spiraling in a scream of incest,
the impatient dog can be heard
over the strain of concealed silence.

BURNING GRASS

The two of them are at it again.
My two helpers out in the field.
Chainsaw in hand and a tank of gas.
They are systematically burning the whole field.
The weather has been so dry
that I fear the whole place will go up in flames.
But these guys have it under control.
They place some gasoline on a stick
and burn in a semi-circle.
They leave gashes in the earth
as large as cornfield rings.
A bird's shadow looks over them.
I sit in my little Pueblo,
smoke undulating around the room.
It wafts across the photos of my wife and child.
It sears the drapes and leaves its scent
among the fibres.
It dances to the sweet music coming out of my tiny radio.
This is Taos at 7000 feet.
Two men burning grass in a field.
Music serenading the silent room
and the longing cry of words from your lover.

Things That Are Wonderful

A pregnant kiss.
A yellow rose in a salon.
A cup of coffee on the highway.
A belief in love.
Soft music on the radio.
A freshly laid hardwood floor.
A working septic system.
Detangling madness.
First smile of a new-born.
Having a full tank of gas.
A new pair of Levi's cords.
A new pair of underwear.
Having a hairdresser you can trust.
Having a lawyer you can trust.
Having anyone you can trust.

In a Moment's Breath

I knew a man who could see in the dark,
who believed that he could fly through the sky
and could visit graves from his past.
I once knew a man who could speak a thousand tongues,
could love like a prince,
and could clothe himself as does an emperor.
He believed all of this.
I knew him well.
He visited our Mission from time to time.
Tired of the cold.
Tired of wandering around waiting for a room to open.
He believed all these things.
With each pill that I gave him,
with each condoned handful,
he found it more difficult to see in the dark.
He could barely walk,
and failed to visit the graves for weeks.
His speech deterred into a vague grunt.
His lust for love suffered.
He hadn't been with anyone in over a year.
As for his clothes,
they kept getting more and more worn.
His face became darkened by fright
and then when the pills had worn off he said:
"I will one day see again.
I will be clothed in pearls and rubies.
I will command the night of a thousand honeymoons.
I will speak to all I meet.
I will . . ."
With his small sack over his shoulder
he left,
and I haven't seen him since.

Continental Breakfast

Loads of day-old doughnuts.
Cereal in plastic cases.
Bagels cut almost clear through.
Toaster so hot that bread burns
the little plastic plates.
Cream cheese melts in a storm.
A wise lady sits smiling.
Would you like some coffee?
You can tell she is proud of her filter skills.
She mastered the acidic tones,
well-placed with two ex-husbands roaming the land.
Akron, Ohio her birthplace.
Ending up in California.
Don't we all end up in California?
It is a State that settles
at the bottom of snow-globes
in Niagara Falls.
A couple of shakes and you get shot on the highway.
A couple more shakes and your car breaks down,
and the madness that was once settled at the bottom
floats all willy-nilly across the smog-filled skies.
Now she sits nursing an ankle,
her boss but another barking manager no doubt bred
 in a tube in the Research Triangle of Raleigh-Durham.
She tells me how to survive hurricanes in a trailer park;
speaks of leaving the windows open just so
to keep the pressure constant.
I've been around the block face
with friends,
crooked lawyers,
husbands from Nantucket, and kids from the moon.
She nurses that foot
while I sip my orange juice,
both of us squinting
from that early morning,
fluorescent glare.

Breast
II

Hope is the thing with
feathers
That perches in the soul
And sings the tune without
the words
And never stops at all.

— *Emily Dickinson*

Sorrow

I can't remember
the last time I cried.
I can't remember
the last time I fucked.
I can't remember
the face of my mentally ill mother.
I can't remember
the smell of our backyard.
I can't remember
the name of my cat.
I can't remember
the last drink.
I can't remember
prayers from church.
I can't remember
the price of my father's funeral.
I can't remember
what they served to eat.
I can't remember
the signed guest list.
I can't remember
the name of the pills
my mother took.
I can't remember
the radiation room.
I can't remember
the licence plate number
of my last car.
I can't remember.
I can't remember
how many months
they gave my grandmother to live.
I can't remember
my lover's skin.
I can't remember
my brother's next court date.

I can't remember
the last time I attended a class.
I can't remember
how to swim.
I can't remember
how to steal an old car.
I can't remember
the name of Lincoln's assassin.
I can't remember
the number of dead in Vietnam.
I can't remember
the last fondle.
I can't remember
the morning we found her.
I can't remember
the ambulance and police officers.
I can't remember
reading the eulogy.
I can't remember
the last time I slept well.
I can't remember.
I just can't
remember . . .

A BASKET OF DISTRESS

I knew that it would happen like this.
I hear the clouds of kestrels circling.
The leaving.
The solitude.
The nights filled will small banshees
making minute noises in the night.
I hear the Navajo drum beats;
wind conveys soft melody of distance.
It crosses vast courses of land.
It seeds in the garden
beside a tinder wheel and toad.
It is ready to be planted
by the unending, undying hands
of a woman who caresses the ground
as she once did her lover.
A basket of tools – her equipment
to dig lust deeper;
it lets spindly flowers grow
wanting but sun.

Fallen Angel

It has see-through wings,
a shade of purple onion
gliding across the screams of hysteria.
A cat breathes its ominous breath,
wheezing away a telling existence.
Soft pines cuddle clouds
and play castanet elixirs to the moon.
Within this cauldron of misplaced mania,
letters of regret keep forming in the letter-box.
They are written in long hand,
an almost forgotten form of art;
messages relayed of crushed alliances
and fetid realities.
Once you brush against the mentally ill,
she coils around your helpless mind
as smooth as a crabby electric eel.
One primitive move and a shock
to spell all shocks.
You really can't blame them
for they learned the careful caress of electricity
from broken down asylums
littered across our landscape.
A few buildings set back,
gates and nail-clipped lawns
the only distance between a crater of rage
and understanding.
Fallen angel dips her wings at Hershey's.
Chocolate hardens.
Impossible to fly.
Tears of regret are shed,
as the frenzied crowd of forgiveness
batters all sense
and coughs up chunks
of half-eaten wings.
They say
it tastes like chicken.

It is morning

Yes, it has finally come.
Dawn full of dogs taunting the last rays of light.
It is in the cool breeze that friendships
are made with the infinite;
they are released as are a batch of doves,
culled to perfection as their wings garner
outer extremes of hope.
This small yet dignified bird,
wholly consumed by the pack
awaiting death silently alone.
This distant shadow
must inevitably come.
Many panic beyond comprehension
holding onto the body as if it were
a timeless artifact.
But it isn't.
Time will soon take us –
soon in the face of signaled prosperity.
I knew as a child all I could hope for
was to get older;
to get my gray hairs
and rock on the porch,
telling stories and tales to grandchildren.
My views haven't changed
only become more honed.
I see the beauty that is now
and bask in its glorious essence.
Having a wife with child
is the most fragile of feelings for a man.
It is the inner need for continuation
that causes great anxiety.
When the first cry of the child is heard,
a release of the inescapable is completed
and tears of absolution flow.
I will always remember those tears.
I will always remember her cry.

It is morning
and birds are singing.
Dogs are barking away the last of the night.
It is in this cocoon of a Pueblo
that I see your vociferous face,
as the light of kindness
heals wounds of longing.

A SILENT PHONE

I remember it vividly.
Going into the hospital.
My mother knows just where to park,
always the same space at the end of the garage.
Her footsteps would echo
as we would walk in silence.
I remember waiting for the elevator,
the smile my mom would give to the next person,
our floor number being pressed.
I remember the nurses station.
Always fresh flowers
sitting in their little holders,
as children in a choir.
I remember the room.
Smell of illness.
Slight click of oxygen from a mask.
I remember the ripped, white sheet
and how it would drape over his small body.
He would attempt to raise his hand
but it would fall in a troubled silence.
She lifted the mask
and he uttered the words,
I love you.
I will never forget the sound.
It came as if from the back of the throat,
a kind of flash as if someone was drowning,
but I knew what I had seen.
I knew he was suffering.
My mom would fiddle with the sheets
as the doctor would enter,
and it was then that I was asked to wait in the hall.
The chairs were always too big.
My feet barely touched the ground.
Without wanting to,
my feet would swing
to some distant rhythm.

I remember the steps back to the parking lot.
Slam of the car door.
I knew then it was the last time I would see my father.
I knew then that the shell was breaking and it wouldn't be long.
For the next week I stayed at a friend's house
as my mother took up the vigil.
She stayed until the end,
until the doctor came in and touched his hands
and told her it won't be long now.
I remember her tears that first night,
the pastor coming over
and wanting her to take something to sleep.
I remember going to the washroom in the night
and seeing light in her room.
It was now *her* room.
She sat up in bed,
her tears welting her face
and said:
"I'm just waiting for that phone to ring.
I just want him on the other end.
Please, please, please ring."
I tucked her in and closed the door,
went to my room
and filled my pillow with gentle tears.

I can smile

I can smile at funerals,
the homeless,
the bomb dropping on innocents,
price of gas,
lies of the new president,
lies of the weather girl,
autopsies,
thimbles of blood,
pre-cut salmon,
long prison sentences,
delayed orgasms,
handcuffs used effectively,
dandruff,
a drunk,
a heroin addict looking for a fix,
a plane crash,
a spit in the gutter,
a messy divorce,
a table full of blood,
a coffee cup full of pus.
I can smile
because when I don't,
I weep in translucent despair.

A Sunday Afternoon

A Swedish ballad
plays on the stereo;
death is mentioned,
once or twice.
Leonard Cohen would smile.
I have just finished doing the dishes.
I had dropped a Kleenex;
it now looks like swirling ghosts
staining the sink.
A pile of dripping dishes.
Incense burning away the afternoon.
My wife and child are off visiting.
I couldn't cope with the smiles today
or *where are you going . . .?*
Instead, I swallow some drops
of canned apple juice,
look out of the dusty Spring windows
and watch the wind caress
both pines and water.
Death is echoing around the room.
A tiny waltz.
Well danced.
Applauded.
Bags of pellets are in a pile
waiting to be burned.
It's too warm today.
Maybe tomorrow.
Guitar ekes its resistance.
It plays minor chords
that are sullenly found
between sadness and despair.
I think it's time to pet the cat.
Yes,
I know
that it's time
to pet the cat.

Pink fluorescent legs

I stepped off the plane
at Raleigh-Durham International,
smell of airport and nursing stations to the left.
Progressive, I thought.
I then saw a little four-year-old girl
with pink fluorescent legs.
Her crutches matched the limbs.
There wasn't any resentment in those eyes,
as if the world owed her.
It was a small child
hobbling with dignity.
In Europe,
that same child would be whisked away
to some country home to be cured.
But there is no cure.
It was decided in the womb
that legs weren't a necessity for this one.
Instead of hiding in a darkened wood,
they are celebrated here in Raleigh.
Those two legs,
reflective stickers seen for miles;
a memory full of passion,
to live fully with what you are given.

Wings

All goes onward and outward,
Nothing collapses
And to die is different from
What anyone supposes
And luckier.

— *Walt Whitman*

Under a Blue Sheet

Wind lifts the edges.
Toes move slowly.
Mattress softly creaks.
Lingerie in a heap.
Sharpening light of morning.
On a wave
of remembered passion,
the song of penetration
lingers
under a blue,
moist sheet.

MATERNITY LEAVE

Lying in a heap.
Eating chocolates until noon.
Not lifting a finger in the kitchen.
Refusing to do dishes.
Full control of the remote.
Forgetting to buy groceries.
Forgetting the keys to the house.
Forgetting almost everything –
and that's just the father to be.

Daisy filled with tears

Flowers are bought for the young;
they are often bought for the old.
They linger at weddings
and lie quite still on coffins at funerals.
In fact, flowers have adorned
hair, lapels, and the romantic teeth
of an enamored lover.
Flowers are everywhere,
almost as numerous as the latest
scratch and sniff sticker.
Flowers are everywhere.
They cover the maypole.
They sneak up on stage divas
in their dressing rooms.
They slide across the ice
at skating competitions;
and if you're lucky,
only if you're truly lucky,
will you get a chance
to see a flower pressed
by your own child.

In the Office

Baby pictures stare from
lightly coloured walls.
Smell of birth still fresh.
Scent of fear present
but subsiding.
Piled pamphlets telling all.
Videos to turn young couples' stomachs.
Promise of classes to come.
A home birth awaits.
A child twiddles thumbs
waiting for the day,
waiting for the surrender.
Biology will spread her giant
butterfly wings,
producing the living –
those thin, seasoned breaths.
Heartbeats on the rise.
Country music swirls
behind the Thank You plants.
A computer jams.
Children's toys in a pile.
There's a slight stain
on one of the chairs,
but it's a home –
a place to realize the agony
and share in the natural process
of pain.
With medical aids on the ready,
a ceiling fan on low,
we'll wait in the faint colour of fall
for another.

Awaiting children

Pine needles fall
after dusk.
Sunshine crawls through
stained bark.
Secrets muffled
underneath calm water.
Distant cry of a tied dog.
Wind rattles rusty oars.
Flashlights confess stained lovers.
Idle chairs sit
mournfully by the lake,
waiting for a chorus
of untainted laughter.
Waiting for a gift.
Thanking the selection,
and praying for survival
between thin labour breaths.

A CHILD'S HEARTBEAT

I felt your skin against me this morning.
I knew that I would be leaving.
You knew nothing,
only pulling out your favourite book for another read.
I made up the story again,
giving a twist so it wouldn't feel old.
There was something different this morning.
You nuzzled close.
Accustomed to space,
I let you wander in the threshold of safety.
We read by the fire.
Our backs were to the lake,
sun over our shoulders.
We read in that sunlight;
your father holding back the agonizing scream,
while carefully and gently
rubbing your tangled hair.

For Emilia

I know that you have taught me
to change a naked child.
You have been kind not to scream
at my fumbling hands.
You have given your father
a sense of hope,
as the disjointed fingers of incest
beckon inside my thin skull
whenever the first drops of a bath
are released.

Pulling a sleigh

I didn't know the laughter of a child
could bring about seizures.
I didn't know that giggles
could echo off of one-hundred-year-old pine trees.
I didn't know snow could reduce stress.
I didn't know that stories could be good
after a fifth consecutive reading.
I didn't know that what goes in
must eventually come out.
I didn't know that a baby's smile
could defrost a fridge.
I didn't know that napping in the afternoon
gives vivid dreams.
I didn't know that Welcome Wagon organizers
all seem the same.
I didn't know that chopping wood
can fascinate a one-year-old.
I didn't know that just last year my life would totally change.
I now know that children ease your way
into growing old with dignity.
May she appreciate the grey hair
of a twenty-nine-year-old.

In a Chinese Buffet

Wheeling my weary child to the table,
I smell the scent of fried chicken,
scant chow mein and
clouds of wonton soup.
She is in a stroller,
bought by my grandmother.
It cost enough dough
that she could have purchased
a car in her day.
Whatever makes you happy.
I'm just trying to help.
My baby is sleeping;
red markings around her lips,
calming reminder of another tattered soother.
The place is almost empty.
It's 3:30 p.m.
Did I mention that it was a buffet?
At 4:00 p.m., dinner prices go into effect.
The only difference between dinner and lunch
are the crab legs.
They are doused with butter,
soaked through as thoroughly as the top layer
of buttered popcorn.
My stomach is growling.
I am hungry.
My wife stumbles from the table and approaches
the three, overflowing islands.
An elderly gentleman
with a two-legged cane
is making his way down the aisle.
His wife full of commitment,
helps him place one foot
in front of the other.
They aren't here for the specials;
they come when there are less crowds.
He limps towards the baby carriage.

My daughter is still sucking that soother.
Let me see the baby.
He stables himself and looks in;
nothing in me takes offense.
The scent of fear is non-existent.
He coughs forth an honest,
"Good luck, kid."
He grabs hold of the freshly wiped cane
and proceeds to leave the restaurant,
leave his childhood,
leave his nearing death behind
in those three, kind-hearted and crushing words:
Good luck, kid.

A SOOTHER IN MY POCKET

I reached into my sunken past
and retrieved your soother.
I didn't know that your small lips
and Superman piece of plastic could be so tender.
I am at the gates of Graceland,
scrolls of millions of visitors carving the wall;
sighs of longing filling the tour bus.
Complaints of:
I liked the tour better when they had a person
to show you around.
From the back someone adds:
I liked it better when Elvis was around . . .
I found out about your existence just a few short years ago.
I was so scared to be a numbskull father.
I still am.
I dream for the day
when I can pick you up off the floor
and hold you against my skin.
I love you, little one.
A soother in my pocket
at the gates of Graceland.

My Daniel

I feel your little hands in the incubator.
I know you are there,
inside the haze of rapid heartbeats
exploding to 270.
Yet you look out,
as if to say I've lived with this inside the womb.
I've seen the shaded light
and felt the pain of being pricked
by an IV in my skull.
Your tiny body shudders
as medicine flushes into your slim veins.
You look out,
not judging,
just staring in a lucid and understanding cradle.
I know the pain that you are feeling.
This is the same hospital
where I almost lost my leg to cancer,
where for a week and a half
they had a social worker talk to me about a one-legged life.
She was kind and compassionate;
all the necessities to keep back tears
until she had left the room.
And they did come.
Usually deep into the night
when moonless and dark.
The IV dripped its drip.
Machines that go *ping*.
Now I'm back in that same hospital.
The one where my dying father came to read
Grade Nine stories for English class
so I could catch up
and wouldn't be left behind.
I didn't have the heart to tell him
that the train had already left.
His consenting cancer
and my mother's suicide

cured that path.
Now I sit in a mostly uncomfortable chair
and watch those machines that go *ping*.
They are monitoring a life.
Daniel.
My son.
Lying in that bed made of steel
by Defasco Union employees;
a volunteer group purchased incubator,
and a room named after a miracle.
They do happen,
these miracles.
Little Daniel.
When I see your eyes,
I know that you are fighting.
I know that the dogs barking are at bay
and that I'll have the courage to hold you
with all of those tubes.
My eyes close on tears
as I chase away another wave.
Monitoring.
Both parent and child.
An indestructible union.

An eagle's wing

Through the sky it flows,
wing of an eagle circling,
looking for a place to land.
Finding a branch.
A break.
He can see the landfill site
just beyond the next crest.
An intermittent fire burns in the distance.
A small boy is being wheeled by his parents.
They stop and periodically kiss
to remind them of love and attrition.
The little boy looks at everything,
taking it all in as if he were a small conch shell.
They continue to kiss,
his leg swinging, urging a continuation of their journey.
The eagle sees a forest of trailer homes.
He can almost hear the laughter and pain from his perch.
Screams are mixed with the joys of giggling.
Satellite dishes shine upwards to the sky.
They follow the distance between clouds and stars.
The eagle gathers up his fragile wing for
a stray bullet had hit him.
He flaps and flies to that place
just beyond the Sierra.

Quest for Absolution

Sequestered in the mountains of deceit,
I know that the path of regulars is distant.
It is folded on passes filled with eagles
who guard the entrance.
People are felled by lightning flashes.
Bombs dropped in unison,
singing as loudly as caged birds
in a Parisian sitting room.
To know this reign of terror,
this site of pure torture;
the cleft of unsightly damage.
This is what the mountains call *secret*.
This is the fallen camp of defenders
that cloud their cover when another satellite
passes into view.
They hide their weapons
and hold onto the solemn prayer
of not being seen.
I didn't see all of this from the road,
only along the past of my marsupial plain.
It is in the deviant act of reconciliation
that Indians were trod to death
and entered the largest reserve ever –
that of our National Prisons.
"Beware of Picking Up Hitchhikers" signs
litter the highway.
One can still hear the faint chant of the booked and beaten.
It is in this strand of greying full hair
that messages of peace and unity are uttered.
They come flowing through a burst dam.
Floods effective.
Tricked by our ears.
All that can be heard are the solemn words:
May peace of Blue Mountains fly above eagles
and roar over the coloured cloud of forever.

Singing the song

Up in the tree,
a bird sings to the wind.
It is a gentle wind
that comes out of the South
and blows the leaves.
I used to know this wind
when I was a child,
when my parents were alive
and the television was still black and white.
I remember sitting on the frontyard,
underneath that tree.
The same one
that in a fit of strangeness
my mother cut down
so it would be easier to mow the lawn.
I used to sit under those blossoming branches
and see the sky over our neighbour's roof.
All the little aerials collecting something from the sky.
All of those family rooms filled with children and parents
not saying a word to each other.
Dad moving off the couch to change the channel
if things got too slow.
What has happened since then?
Now the colour is vivid.
A converter allows you to flip simultaneously
through the tens of channels.
Something was lost that day
when the tree was cut down –
the same way as something was lost
when you failed to see your father
get up off the couch,
to change the channel
to something better.

Acknowledgments

I would like to thank the Canada Council and Ontario Arts Council for funding and The Helene Wurlitzer Foundation of New Mexico for giving me time and a quiet space to complete this collection. Many of the poems were written in Taos, New Mexico at The Helene Wurlitzer Foundation in my little Pueblo. Thank you to Michael A. Knight, Foundation Director for accommodating me. I was to "just write" . . .

I want to thank Boheme Press with the editorial decisions and Max Maccari for his kindness. Both were superb and unexpected in this changing world. There is still hope. I want to thank Matt Firth again for his relentless support of my work. Shannon Babcock is a diligent believer in this collection. Her incredible insight gave me the light to form the divisions. Thank you Suzanne A. Marsden for being a truly gifted artist and superb friend. It is always an honour to work with you. And to Midori Okada for the Japanese character references.

Without Victoria this collection would not have been possible. I was told once that I got the "calm" one. When my vernacular storm of incomprehension spins, her light leads the way to sanity. I am eternally grateful. Thank you both Emilia and Daniel for giving me an opportunity to be "Daddy." You've made my life complete. Through you all I've learned there is a place called *family*.